REAL-WORLD EVIDENCE

A Guide for Researchers and Practitioners

Dr Essam Abdelhakim

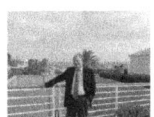

Copyright © 2024 Dr Essam Abdelhakim

All rights reserved

The characters and events portrayed in this book are fictitious. Any similarity to real persons, living or dead, is coincidental and not intended by the author.

No part of this book may be reproduced, or stored in a retrieval system, or transmitted in any form or by any means, electronic, mechanical, photocopying, recording, or otherwise, without express written permission of the publisher.

Cover design by: Art Painter
Library of Congress Control Number: 2018675309
Printed in the United States of America

CONTENTS

Title Page
Copyright
Chapter 1: Introduction to Real-World Evidence — 1
Chapter 2: Understanding Real-World Data (RWD) — 8
Chapter 3: Methodologies in Real-World Evidence Studies — 16
Chapter 4: Conducting Real-World Evidence Studies — 25
Chapter 5: RWE in Regulatory Decision-Making — 34
Chapter 6: RWE in Health Economics and Outcomes Research — 42
Chapter 7: Real-World Evidence in Drug Development and Post-Market Surveillance — 50
Chapter 8: Challenges and Limitations of Real-World Evidence — 58
Chapter 9: The Future of Real-World Evidence — 64
Chapter 10: Case Studies in Real-World Evidence Applications — 71
Appendices — 84
About The Author — 93

CHAPTER 1: INTRODUCTION TO REAL-WORLD EVIDENCE

Definition and Distinction Between Clinical Trial Data and Real-World Evidence

Real-World Evidence (RWE) refers to the clinical evidence derived from the analysis of Real-World Data (RWD), which is collected outside the controlled environment of traditional clinical trials.

RWE is used to assess the effectiveness and safety of treatments in broader, more heterogeneous populations, providing insights into how interventions perform in routine clinical practice, beyond the limited, carefully selected groups in randomized controlled trials (RCTs).

In contrast, **clinical trial data** comes from randomized controlled trials, which are typically conducted in tightly controlled settings with carefully defined inclusion and exclusion criteria. The goal of RCTs is to establish the efficacy of a treatment by isolating it from confounding factors, ensuring that the results are as reliable and scientifically rigorous as possible.

However, these trials often have a limited ability to generalize results to diverse populations, especially those with complex comorbidities or demographic factors that may not have been included in the study.

Key Differences Between Clinical Trial Data and RWE:

- **Study Design**: RCTs are designed with strict protocols, randomization, and control groups to minimize bias, while RWE is based on data collected in routine clinical practice, often without randomized control.

- **Population**: RCTs usually focus on a homogenous, ideal patient population that meets specific eligibility criteria. In contrast, RWE includes a broader, more diverse range of patients, reflecting real-world complexities such as multiple comorbidities and variations in treatment adherence.
- **Data Collection**: RCTs generate data through predefined endpoints and measurements within a controlled setting. RWE, on the other hand, gathers data from varied sources like electronic health records, insurance claims, and patient-reported outcomes over extended periods.
- **Outcome Measures**: While RCTs focus on clinical endpoints like survival rates or disease-specific measures, RWE often includes broader outcomes, such as quality of life, healthcare resource utilization, and long-term safety, which may be difficult to measure in controlled trials.

Types of Real-World Data (RWD)

Real-World Data (RWD) is the backbone of RWE, and it encompasses any health-related data that is collected outside of the controlled environment of clinical trials.

Some of the primary types of RWD include:

1. **Electronic Health Records (EHRs)**: These are digital versions of patients' paper charts and contain detailed information about their medical history, diagnoses, treatments, medications, lab results, and other clinical data. EHRs are one of the most valuable sources of RWD, as they allow for the tracking of individual patient data over time, across multiple healthcare

settings.

2. **Insurance Claims Data**: This data includes information from health insurance companies about the treatments patients receive, including prescriptions, procedures, diagnoses, and healthcare costs. It provides a large-scale overview of how healthcare is utilized and can be used to study treatment patterns, outcomes, and cost-effectiveness.

3. **Patient Registries**: Patient registries are databases that collect information about patients with specific diseases or conditions. These registries are particularly useful for studying rare diseases or conditions with long-term outcomes, as they provide a repository of clinical data that can be analyzed for trends, treatment responses, and real-world efficacy.

4. **Wearable Devices and Mobile Health Applications**: With the advent of digital health technologies, data from wearable devices (such as fitness trackers, heart rate monitors, glucose meters, etc.) and mobile health apps are becoming increasingly valuable in RWE research. These devices can provide continuous, real-time data on patients' physiological status, activity levels, and adherence to treatment protocols.

5. **Social Media and Patient-Reported Outcomes (PROs)**: Social media platforms and online patient forums can serve as a source of data on patients' experiences, attitudes, and perceptions about their diseases and treatments. Additionally, patient-reported outcomes (PROs) are self-reported data from patients about their health status, symptoms, and quality of life, which can be collected via surveys, mobile apps, or other digital platforms.

Sources of RWD

Each of the sources of RWD mentioned above offers unique insights into patient outcomes, treatment patterns, and healthcare resource utilization:

1. **Electronic Health Records (EHR)**: EHRs are a comprehensive source of clinical data, allowing researchers to track patient diagnoses, treatments, lab results, and outcomes over time. The widespread adoption of EHRs has revolutionized the ability to conduct observational studies and follow patients longitudinally.

2. **Insurance Claims Data**: Claims data is often used in health economics studies to assess the cost-effectiveness of treatments and interventions, as it provides detailed billing and reimbursement data. Claims data can also be used to monitor post-market safety and identify treatment patterns across large, diverse patient populations.

3. **Patient Registries**: Patient registries are particularly useful for studying diseases with lower incidence rates, where traditional clinical trials may not provide enough data. For example, registries for rare diseases, oncology, or specific types of cardiovascular disease provide valuable insights into treatment effectiveness and safety across a broad range of patients.

4. **Wearable Devices and Mobile Health**: These tools offer real-time data on patients' daily activities, medication adherence, and vital signs. Wearable devices can provide continuous, objective data on disease progression, physical functioning, and response to therapy, making them a powerful tool in longitudinal RWE studies.

5. **Social Media and PROs**: While not always structured or standardized, social media and patient-reported data offer qualitative insights into patient experiences,

satisfaction, and symptom burden. These sources can complement traditional clinical data by providing a patient-centered perspective on health and treatment outcomes.

Key Differences Between Randomized Controlled Trials (Rcts) And Real-World Studies

*While both RCTs and RWE are integra*l to advancing medical knowledge, they have distinct differences that influence their design, execution, and outcomes:

1. **Control and Randomization**: RCTs use randomization to allocate treatments and control for confounding variables, ensuring that the results are unbiased and reproducible. In contrast, RWE studies are often observational and may not have random assignment, making them more vulnerable to confounding factors, such as treatment selection bias.

2. **Study Population**: RCTs tend to focus on a highly selective group of participants who meet specific inclusion and exclusion criteria, limiting the generalizability of the findings. RWE, by utilizing data from diverse patient populations, can provide insights that are more representative of the real-world clinical setting.

3. **External Validity**: The primary strength of RCTs lies in their internal validity (i.e., the ability to establish causal relationships between interventions and outcomes). However, their external validity, or generalizability to the broader population, is often limited. RWE studies, on the other hand, have higher external validity because they reflect the complexity and diversity of real-world patient populations.

4. **Outcome Measures**: RCTs typically focus on

predefined, clinical endpoints, such as survival rates, disease-free intervals, or other objective measures of treatment success. RWE often includes a wider range of outcomes, including health-related quality of life, patient satisfaction, and healthcare utilization, providing a more holistic view of treatment impacts.

Benefits And Limitations Of Rwe In Clinical Research

Benefits:

1. **Real-World Applicability**: RWE reflects how treatments work in the general population, including patients with comorbidities, polypharmacy, and other characteristics often excluded from clinical trials. This makes RWE particularly valuable in assessing treatment effectiveness in routine clinical practice.

2. **Long-Term Insights**: While RCTs may have limited follow-up periods, RWE can provide long-term data on the safety and efficacy of treatments, helping to monitor post-market outcomes and rare adverse events.

3. **Cost-Effectiveness**: RWE can inform cost-effectiveness analyses by incorporating real-world healthcare resource utilization, treatment adherence, and patient outcomes. This is important for healthcare policymakers and payers when evaluating new treatments or therapies.

4. **Flexibility**: RWE studies can be adapted to various research questions and can incorporate diverse data sources, making them flexible for different types of studies, from observational cohort studies to post-marketing surveillance.

Limitations:

1. **Bias and Confounding**: Since RWE studies are often observational, they are more susceptible to biases and confounding variables compared to RCTs. Researchers must use advanced statistical techniques to adjust for these potential biases.
2. **Data Quality**: The accuracy and completeness of RWD can vary, depending on the source. EHRs, for example, may have missing or inconsistent data, which can affect the validity of RWE studies.
3. **Causal Inference**: While RWE can suggest associations between interventions and outcomes, making definitive causal inferences is more challenging due to the observational nature of the data.
4. **Ethical and Privacy Concerns**: The use of large-scale patient data raises concerns about patient privacy and data security, and researchers must ensure that data is anonymized and that ethical standards are adhered to in all stages of research.

CHAPTER 2: UNDERSTANDING REAL-WORLD DATA (RWD)

Real-World Data (RWD) serves as the foundation for Real-World Evidence (RWE). It encompasses data that reflects the conditions and experiences of patients in everyday clinical practice, outside the controlled environment of clinical trials.

RWD can be collected from a variety of sources, including clinical databases, patient registries, insurance claims data, surveys, and other forms of observational data.

Data Sources: Clinical Databases, Patient Registries, Claims Data, Surveys, And Other Observational Data

1. **Clinical Databases**: Clinical databases are centralized repositories that store patient data collected from various healthcare settings, such as hospitals, outpatient clinics, or specialized healthcare centers. These databases often include detailed clinical information such as diagnoses, laboratory test results, treatments administered, and follow-up outcomes. Examples include Electronic Health Records (EHRs) and clinical trial databases. These sources provide rich, detailed, and longitudinal data that can be used for cohort studies, patient outcome analysis, and safety monitoring.
    - **Strengths**: High granularity of clinical data, long-term follow-up potential.

- **Challenges**: Data consistency, integration of data from multiple sources, and potential gaps in documentation.
2. **Patient Registries**: Patient registries are systematic collections of data about patients with a specific disease or condition. These registries may focus on rare diseases, chronic conditions, or conditions with high unmet medical need. Registries often include demographic information, clinical characteristics, treatment regimens, and patient-reported outcomes.
    - **Strengths**: Ideal for studying rare diseases or conditions with complex treatment regimens. Provides insights into long-term patient outcomes and treatment efficacy in the real world.
    - **Challenges**: Potential for selection bias if the registry is not representative of the broader patient population.
3. **Claims Data**: Claims data is collected from health insurance companies or government payers (e.g., Medicare or Medicaid in the U.S.), which contain information about treatments, procedures, medications, diagnoses, and costs associated with healthcare. This data is typically collected for billing purposes but is widely used in health economics and outcomes research to understand treatment patterns, healthcare costs, and patient outcomes.
    - **Strengths**: Large-scale data, provides insights into healthcare utilization and cost-effectiveness.
    - **Challenges**: Limited clinical detail (e.g., lacks laboratory results or disease severity indicators), potential for errors in coding.
4. **Surveys and Patient-Reported Outcomes (PROs)**:

Surveys and PROs are used to gather information directly from patients about their health status, quality of life, symptoms, treatment satisfaction, and functional outcomes. These data sources provide a patient-centered view that is often missing from clinical data. PROs are especially valuable for understanding the impact of a disease or treatment from the patient's perspective.

- **Strengths**: Provides direct insight into patients' experiences, quality of life, and satisfaction.
- **Challenges**: Risk of recall bias, self-reporting bias, and incomplete data collection.

5. **Other Observational Data**: Other types of observational data may come from sources such as social media platforms, wearable health devices, and mobile apps. These sources can offer real-time, continuous monitoring data and provide insights into patients' lifestyle, adherence to treatments, and disease progression outside of the healthcare setting.

- **Strengths**: Real-time, continuous data collection, capturing behaviors and adherence patterns that are difficult to measure through other means.
- **Challenges**: Data privacy concerns, lack of standardization, and potential for inaccurate or incomplete data.

Data Quality, Validation, And Standardization

The quality of Real-World Data is one of the most critical aspects that affect the reliability and credibility of the resulting Real-World Evidence.

High-quality data ensures that the insights generated are

accurate, reproducible, and actionable.

Below are key considerations for data quality, validation, and standardization:

1. **Data Quality**:
    - **Completeness**: Data should include all relevant variables and patient details, without significant gaps. Missing data can lead to biased results or underrepresentation of important patient outcomes.
    - **Accuracy**: Data should be accurate and correctly represent the clinical situation. Errors in data entry, such as incorrect diagnoses or treatment codes, can skew results.
    - **Consistency**: Data should be consistent across various sources, formats, and platforms. Discrepancies between different data systems may lead to challenges in interpreting the data.
2. **Data Validation**: Validation is the process of ensuring that the data collected is accurate, reliable, and consistent. This can be achieved through:
    - **Cross-referencing**: Validating data by comparing it across different sources (e.g., matching patient data from clinical databases with claims data).
    - **Automated checks**: Using data validation algorithms and software tools to identify and correct errors or inconsistencies in real-time.
    - **Manual review**: Conducting periodic manual reviews of the data to ensure that it adheres to established clinical standards and is free from obvious errors.

3. **Data Standardization**: Standardizing data is essential to ensure that it can be compared across various sources and analyzed efficiently. This involves:
    - **Coding systems**: Using standardized coding systems (e.g., ICD-10 for diagnoses, ATC for drug classifications) to ensure consistency in data representation.
    - **Data formats**: Adopting standardized formats for storing and exchanging data (e.g., HL7 or CDISC standards for clinical trial data).
    - **Data dictionaries**: Creating detailed dictionaries or glossaries that define the terms, variables, and codes used in the data to ensure clarity and consistency across studies.

Types Of Rwd: Prospective Vs. Retrospective, Observational Vs. Interventional

Real-World Data can be classified based on how and when it is collected, and the nature of the research design.

1. **Prospective vs. Retrospective**:
    - **Prospective RWD** refers to data that is collected moving forward in time. Patients are observed in real time, and data are gathered as they receive treatment or experience outcomes. This type of data collection allows for more control over what is recorded and can be designed to answer specific research questions.
        - **Example**: A cohort of patients with a particular disease is followed over several years to assess the long-term

effectiveness of a new drug.
- **Retrospective RWD** refers to data collected from past records or databases. Researchers analyze pre-existing data to explore relationships between treatment and outcomes, without influencing how the data is gathered.
    - **Example**: Analyzing patient charts from several hospitals to study the outcomes of a certain medication over the past five years.

2. **Observational vs. Interventional**:
    - **Observational RWD** refers to data collected without any direct intervention from the researcher. In these studies, patients are observed in their natural setting, receiving standard treatments or experiencing health events as they occur.
        - **Example**: A study of the outcomes of diabetic patients receiving different forms of insulin, where researchers observe and record the treatments patients are already receiving without influencing the choice of therapy.
    - **Interventional RWD** involves actively intervening with patients, such as enrolling them in a specific treatment or altering their standard treatment plan as part of the study. This type of study blurs the line between traditional clinical trials and observational studies.
        - **Example**: A pragmatic clinical trial that compares the effectiveness

of two different blood pressure medications in a general patient population.

Ethical Considerations And Data Privacy Concerns

As Real-World Data often includes sensitive patient information, maintaining patient privacy and adhering to ethical guidelines is essential for the integrity of research and compliance with legal requirements.

1. **Informed Consent**:
    - In traditional clinical trials, participants must give explicit, informed consent before their data can be collected. However, in RWD studies, especially those using historical data or claims data, obtaining informed consent may be more complicated. Researchers must ensure that the data is anonymized and that patients are aware of how their information will be used.
    - **Challenges**: Patients may not always be aware that their data is being used for research purposes, particularly with data from EHRs, claims, or social media.
2. **Data Privacy**:
    - RWD often contains personally identifiable information (PII) and health-related data that must be handled with the utmost care. Laws like the Health Insurance Portability and Accountability Act (HIPAA) in the U.S., and the General Data Protection Regulation (GDPR) in the EU, establish strict guidelines for data protection.
    - **Challenges**: Ensuring that patient data is de-

identified or anonymized to prevent misuse or breaches, while still maintaining enough detail for analysis.

3. **Ethical Approval**:
   - Research involving RWD must still adhere to ethical research guidelines, including review by Institutional Review Boards (IRBs) or Ethics Committees. These bodies ensure that studies are designed to minimize harm, protect patient privacy, and achieve meaningful outcomes.

Data Linkage And Integration Challenges

One of the key challenges in working with Real-World Data is the integration of data from disparate sources, each with its own structure, format, and quality standards.

Data linkage and integration allow researchers to combine different data sets to create a more comprehensive and accurate picture of patient health and treatment outcomes.

CHAPTER 3: METHODOLOGIES IN REAL-WORLD EVIDENCE STUDIES

Real-World Evidence (RWE) is derived from the analysis of Real-World Data (RWD) using a variety of study designs and statistical methodologies.

Study Designs In Rwe Studies

1. **Cohort Studies:**
    - **Definition:** Cohort studies involve following a group (cohort) of individuals over time to assess the outcomes of interest. This design is often used to compare the effects of exposure to a particular treatment, intervention, or risk factor.
    - **Types:**
        - **Prospective Cohort Studies:** Data is collected going forward from a defined starting point. Patients are grouped based on exposure to the treatment or risk factor, and outcomes are measured over time.
        - **Retrospective Cohort Studies:** These studies analyze historical data from patient records to track outcomes from a past exposure.
    - **Strengths:** Cohort studies provide strong

evidence for causality by observing the temporal relationship between exposure and outcome. They are particularly useful when studying long-term effects.
  - **Challenges**: Cohort studies can be resource-intensive and time-consuming, particularly when following patients over extended periods.
2. **Case-Control Studies**:
    - **Definition**: Case-control studies compare patients who have a specific outcome (cases) with those who do not (controls). The goal is to identify exposures or risk factors that are more common in cases than in controls.
    - **Strengths**: Case-control studies are often used for studying rare diseases or conditions and can be conducted more quickly than cohort studies.
    - **Challenges**: They are prone to recall bias, as exposure data is typically collected retrospectively, and matching controls can be difficult. Establishing causality is also challenging because the direction of association between exposure and outcome is less clear.
3. **Cross-Sectional Studies**:
    - **Definition**: Cross-sectional studies collect data at a single point in time to assess the prevalence of an outcome or to compare different groups on certain variables.
    - **Strengths**: They are typically fast and inexpensive to conduct and can provide valuable descriptive data, especially for understanding the burden of disease or

the distribution of characteristics in a population.
- **Challenges**: These studies are limited in their ability to infer causality because they lack temporal information. They only capture associations, not causal relationships.

4. **Pragmatic Trials**:
   - **Definition**: Pragmatic trials are designed to assess the effectiveness of interventions in real-world clinical settings, as opposed to the highly controlled environments of randomized controlled trials (RCTs). These trials often include diverse patient populations and take into account real-world complexities such as co-morbidities, adherence, and socio-economic factors.
   - **Strengths**: Pragmatic trials provide more generalizable results than RCTs, making them highly relevant for real-world clinical decision-making.
   - **Challenges**: They may suffer from greater variability in outcomes due to the inclusion of a broader patient population and lack of strict controls.

Statistical Methodologies In Rwe Studies

To draw reliable conclusions from RWD, researchers must apply rigorous statistical techniques.

Here, we explore the most commonly used statistical methodologies in RWE studies.

1. **Propensity Score Matching**:
   - **Definition**: Propensity score matching is

used to account for selection bias in observational studies. It involves estimating the probability (propensity score) that a patient would receive a particular treatment based on observed characteristics, and then matching patients in the treatment group with those in the control group who have similar propensity scores.
- **Strengths**: Helps reduce confounding by balancing baseline characteristics between treatment groups, mimicking randomization.
- **Challenges**: Matching may not fully eliminate bias if there are unmeasured confounders. The quality of matching depends on the accuracy of the propensity score model.

2. **Regression Models**:
    - **Definition**: Regression analysis is used to assess the relationship between one or more independent variables (e.g., treatment, demographic factors) and a dependent variable (e.g., health outcome). Common regression models in RWE studies include linear regression, logistic regression, and Cox proportional hazards regression.
    - **Strengths**: Allows for adjustment of multiple confounders and estimation of the effect size. Regression models can be extended to handle complex data structures.
    - **Challenges**: Model assumptions must be checked (e.g., linearity, independence of errors), and model selection should be done carefully to avoid overfitting or underfitting.

3. **Survival Analysis:**
   - **Definition:** Survival analysis is used to analyze time-to-event data, such as the time until a patient experiences a specific outcome (e.g., death, disease recurrence, or treatment failure). Key techniques include Kaplan-Meier estimation and Cox proportional hazards models.
   - **Strengths:** Survival analysis is invaluable in analyzing time-to-event outcomes, especially in chronic diseases, where outcomes may occur over long periods.
   - **Challenges:** Censoring (when a patient's event is not observed within the study period) can complicate interpretation, requiring specialized statistical methods.

Advanced Techniques In Rwe Studies

1. **Machine Learning (ML):**
   - **Definition:** Machine learning algorithms are increasingly being applied in RWE studies to uncover complex patterns in large datasets. These algorithms can automatically identify relationships between variables and make predictions based on data. Common methods include decision trees, random forests, and support vector machines (SVM).
   - **Strengths:** ML can handle high-dimensional data and uncover non-linear relationships that may be difficult to detect with traditional statistical methods. It is particularly useful in predicting patient outcomes, treatment responses, and

identifying patient subgroups.
- **Challenges**: Machine learning models can be "black boxes," making them difficult to interpret. Moreover, their performance depends on the quality and quantity of data available.

2. **Artificial Intelligence (AI)**:
   - **Definition**: AI encompasses a broad range of technologies, including deep learning, natural language processing (NLP), and neural networks. AI is used to process large and unstructured datasets such as medical imaging, EHRs, and even unstructured text data from clinical notes.
   - **Strengths**: AI can automate data analysis, improving efficiency and discovering insights that may not be apparent through traditional methods. It can also handle large, unstructured data sources like free-text clinical notes.
   - **Challenges**: AI models require vast amounts of data for training and can be sensitive to data quality. They also pose challenges related to interpretability, ethics, and privacy.

Handling Confounders, Biases, And Missing Data

1. **Confounders**:
   - **Definition**: Confounders are variables that are associated with both the exposure (e.g., treatment) and the outcome, and may distort the true relationship between them.
   - **Methodologies to Address Confounders**:

- **Matching techniques** (e.g., propensity score matching) help balance confounders between treated and untreated groups.
- **Multivariable regression models** can adjust for multiple confounders simultaneously.

2. **Bias:**
    - **Definition**: Bias refers to systematic errors that lead to incorrect conclusions. Common biases in RWE studies include selection bias (due to non-random allocation of treatment) and information bias (due to inaccuracies in data collection or reporting).
    - **Methodologies to Address Bias:**
        - **Instrumental variable analysis** can help control for unmeasured confounding by using variables that influence the treatment but are not directly related to the outcome.
        - **Sensitivity analysis** can help assess how robust the results are to different assumptions and biases.

3. **Missing Data:**
    - **Definition**: Missing data occurs when information is absent for some patients in the dataset. This is common in RWD studies due to incomplete records or non-responses in surveys.
    - **Methods for Handling Missing Data:**
        - **Multiple imputation** creates several plausible values for missing data and combines results to estimate

the final outcome.
- **Complete case analysis** excludes patients with missing data, although this can introduce bias if the missingness is not random.

Sensitivity Analysis and Robustness Checks

1. **Sensitivity Analysis**:
   - **Definition**: Sensitivity analysis is used to assess how sensitive the results are to changes in model assumptions, data handling techniques, and analytical choices. It helps identify whether the conclusions drawn from a study hold up under different scenarios.
   - **Methods**:
     - Varying the inclusion/exclusion criteria for the study population.
     - Testing different methods for handling missing data (e.g., imputation vs. complete case analysis).
     - Using different statistical models or regression techniques.

2. **Robustness Checks**:
   - **Definition**: Robustness checks are used to verify the stability and reliability of the findings by testing the results under various conditions.
   - **Methods**:
     - Applying alternative statistical techniques to ensure consistent results.
     - Performing subgroup analyses to

examine whether the findings hold across different patient populations or disease subgroups.

CHAPTER 4: CONDUCTING REAL-WORLD EVIDENCE STUDIES

Conducting Real-World Evidence (RWE) studies requires a thorough and systematic approach to ensure that the research is meaningful, reliable, and applicable to clinical practice.

Defining Research Questions And Hypotheses For Rwe Studies

1. **Importance of a Clear Research Question**:
    - The research question is the foundation of any study. In RWE, these questions are often more focused on understanding the effectiveness, safety, and long-term outcomes of treatments in broader, heterogeneous populations, outside the controlled environment of clinical trials.
    - Examples of typical RWE research questions include:
        - "What is the real-world effectiveness of drug X in patients with comorbidities?"
        - "How do treatment patterns vary in patients with chronic conditions like diabetes or heart disease?"
        - "What are the long-term health outcomes for patients using a particular therapy compared to a

conventional one?"
2. **Formulating Hypotheses**:
    - Based on the research question, hypotheses are developed to test the presumed relationships between exposure (e.g., a treatment or intervention) and outcomes (e.g., disease progression or quality of life).
    - Hypotheses in RWE studies often take into account the broad variability of real-world populations. For instance:
        - **Null Hypothesis (H0)**: "There is no significant difference in health outcomes between patients treated with Drug A and those treated with Drug B."
        - **Alternative Hypothesis (Ha)**: "Patients treated with Drug A experience significantly better health outcomes compared to those treated with Drug B."
3. **Refining the Research Question**:
    - Ensure that the research question is specific, measurable, and feasible within the context of available real-world data. It should address practical clinical issues and be designed in a way that reflects the realities of patient care in the general population.

Study Design And Protocol Development For Rwe Studies

1. **Study Design Selection**:
    - **Observational vs. Interventional**: While

RWE studies often focus on observational designs (e.g., cohort studies, case-control studies), some interventional studies may also be conducted (e.g., pragmatic trials).

- **Prospective vs. Retrospective**: Depending on available data and resources, you must decide whether the study will be prospective (data is collected going forward) or retrospective (analyzing pre-existing data). Prospective studies are ideal for minimizing bias but require more resources.
- **Cohort Studies**: These studies follow a group of patients who share common characteristics (e.g., same treatment regimen or disease condition) to evaluate outcomes over time.
- **Case-Control Studies**: In these studies, patients with a specific outcome (case group) are compared to those without it (control group) to identify factors associated with the outcome.
- **Pragmatic Trials**: These trials aim to test interventions in real-world clinical settings, capturing the diversity of patient characteristics and healthcare delivery.

2. **Protocol Development**:
    - The protocol outlines the detailed methodology for the RWE study and serves as a roadmap for the entire research process. It includes the research question, hypotheses, study design, data sources, statistical methods, and ethical considerations.
    - A well-structured protocol should define:

- **Study Population**: Criteria for inclusion and exclusion of patients (age, disease stage, treatment history, etc.).
- **Outcomes**: The primary and secondary outcomes, such as mortality, disease progression, or quality of life.
- **Sample Size**: Statistical calculations to determine how many patients are needed to achieve reliable results.
- **Statistical Methods**: The analytical approaches for handling data and testing hypotheses.
- **Ethical Considerations**: Ensuring patient confidentiality, consent, and appropriate handling of sensitive data.

3. **Regulatory Approvals**:
    - Depending on the country and type of data used, regulatory bodies may require approval before the study begins. This includes Institutional Review Board (IRB) approval for human subjects research, especially if new data is being collected or sensitive data is used.

Selection Of Appropriate Data Sources And Data Extraction

1. **Data Source Selection**:
    - Identifying the right data sources is critical to ensuring the validity and reliability of the study results. Common sources of Real-

World Data (RWD) include:
- **Electronic Health Records (EHRs)**: EHRs provide detailed clinical information, including diagnosis, treatment, and patient outcomes, making them a primary source for RWE studies.
- **Insurance Claims Data**: These datasets include billing information, diagnostic codes, and prescriptions, which can be valuable for assessing treatment patterns, healthcare utilization, and outcomes in large populations.
- **Patient Registries**: Disease-specific registries capture detailed information on patients' health status, treatments, and outcomes. These are particularly useful for studying rare diseases.
- **Wearable Devices and Digital Health Data**: Devices such as fitness trackers, smartwatches, and other wearables generate real-time data on health metrics like activity levels, heart rate, and sleep patterns, which can be analyzed for health trends and outcomes.
- **Social Media and Patient Forums**: Although less conventional, social media platforms and patient forums can provide insight into patient experiences, unmet needs, and real-world treatment adherence.

2. **Data Extraction**:
    - Once data sources are identified, the next step is data extraction. This process involves pulling the relevant data points (e.g., patient demographics, clinical history, treatment exposure, and outcomes) from diverse systems.
    - **Data Integration**: It is often necessary to integrate data from different sources (e.g., EHR, claims data) to create a more comprehensive dataset. Data linkage strategies, such as matching patients across databases based on identifiers like patient IDs or demographic characteristics, may be employed.

Data Cleaning, Transformation, And Preparation

1. **Data Cleaning**:
    - Raw data collected from real-world sources often contains errors, inconsistencies, and missing values that need to be addressed before analysis. Data cleaning involves:
        - **Identifying and correcting errors** in data, such as incorrect patient identifiers, inconsistent diagnostic codes, or invalid dates.
        - **Handling missing data**: Methods such as imputation (filling in missing values) or complete case analysis (removing records with missing data) are used, depending on the type and amount of missing information.

- **Outlier detection**: Identifying extreme values that might distort the analysis, such as implausibly high or low measurements of certain variables.

2. **Data Transformation**:
    - In order to analyze the data effectively, it often needs to be transformed. This might involve:
        - **Categorizing continuous variables** (e.g., age groups or BMI categories) to simplify analysis.
        - **Creating composite scores** (e.g., Charlson Comorbidity Index) to assess comorbidity burden.
        - **Standardizing data** to ensure consistency across different data sources (e.g., harmonizing diagnostic codes from multiple systems).

3. **Data Preparation**:
    - Once cleaned and transformed, the data is prepared for analysis. This includes ensuring that all variables are properly coded, outcomes are defined clearly, and that data is organized into the correct structure for statistical analysis (e.g., long vs. wide formats for longitudinal data).
    - **Data Validation**: Cross-checking the prepared dataset with source documents (e.g., clinical records or registry entries) to ensure accuracy and completeness.

Methods For Measuring Treatment Outcomes And Health Status In Real-World Settings

1. **Treatment Outcomes:**
   - **Effectiveness**: One of the primary goals of RWE is to assess the effectiveness of a treatment in a real-world setting. This can include:
     - **Survival outcomes** (e.g., overall survival, progression-free survival)
     - **Disease-specific outcomes** (e.g., remission rates, reduction in biomarkers)
     - **Functional outcomes** (e.g., improvement in physical function or mental health)
     - **Quality of Life (QoL)**: The impact of a treatment on a patient's overall well-being, as measured by standardized tools like the EQ-5D or SF-36.
2. **Health Status Measurement:**
   - **Clinical measures**: Direct measures of disease activity, such as blood pressure, cholesterol levels, tumor size, or joint function, are often used to assess health status.
   - **Patient-reported outcomes (PROs)**: PROs capture a patient's perspective on their own health status, including symptoms, mental health, and treatment satisfaction. These are particularly important in chronic disease management and in assessing the burden of

disease.
- **Healthcare utilization**: RWD often includes information on hospitalizations, emergency room visits, medication adherence, and outpatient visits, which can help assess the broader impact of treatment.

3. **Measurement Tools**:
   - Tools such as validated questionnaires, scales, and biomarkers are commonly used to assess treatment outcomes and health status in RWE studies. These tools help ensure consistency and reliability across different study settings.

CHAPTER 5: RWE IN REGULATORY DECISION-MAKING

Real-World Evidence (RWE) is increasingly playing a pivotal role in shaping regulatory decision-making processes across various health authorities, such as the U.S. Food and Drug Administration (FDA), the European Medicines Agency (EMA), and other global regulators.

As clinical research evolves, regulatory agencies have started to recognize the value of RWE in supplementing traditional randomized controlled trials (RCTs) and contributing to the approval of new therapies, particularly in areas where controlled trials may not be feasible or sufficient.

Role Of Rwe In Regulatory Submissions (Fda, Ema, Etc.)

1. **Increasing Recognition of RWE**:
    - **Regulatory Shift**: Traditionally, regulatory agencies like the FDA and EMA have relied heavily on data from RCTs to approve new drugs and treatments. However, RWE is now being recognized as a valuable complement to these trials, offering insights into how drugs perform in broader, more diverse patient populations under routine clinical conditions.
    - **FDA Initiatives**: The FDA has been a leader in integrating RWE into regulatory processes. The **21st Century Cures Act**

(2016) and the **FDA's Real-World Evidence Program** aim to promote the use of RWE in regulatory decision-making, particularly for post-market surveillance and approving therapies for conditions where traditional trials might be impractical.

- **EMA's Position**: The EMA has also been exploring the use of RWE for decision-making, particularly in cases of therapies for complex diseases or when conducting traditional trials is difficult (e.g., rare diseases, or treatments with long-term outcomes).

2. **Use of RWE in Regulatory Submissions**:
    - **Supplementing Traditional Data**: RWE can provide additional context to clinical trial data, particularly in terms of long-term safety and effectiveness, patient adherence, or the comparative effectiveness of treatments in routine practice. Regulatory agencies may accept RWE in submissions for:
        - **Initial approval**: When existing RCTs may not provide enough evidence for specific subpopulations or long-term outcomes.
        - **Label expansions**: RWE can provide support for expanding the indications of a drug or therapy.
        - **Post-marketing requirements**: For monitoring the safety and effectiveness of a drug once it is approved and available in the market.

3. **Types of Regulatory Submissions**:
    - **New Drug Applications (NDAs)**: The FDA and other regulatory agencies are increasingly considering RWE data as part of NDAs for new drug approvals. For example, RWE can be used to demonstrate a drug's effectiveness across a more diverse population than in traditional trials.
    - **Biologics License Applications (BLAs)**: Similar to NDAs, BLAs for biologics may incorporate RWE, particularly when clinical trials cannot capture real-world conditions.
    - **Abbreviated New Drug Applications (ANDAs)**: In the case of generic drugs, RWE can help demonstrate that a generic drug performs similarly to its branded counterpart in a real-world setting.

Integration Of Rwe Into Clinical Trial Designs

1. **Adaptive Clinical Trial Designs**:
    - **Adaptive Trials**: Adaptive clinical trial designs allow for modifications to the trial protocol based on interim results. RWE can support these trials by providing background data on expected outcomes, patient responses, and healthcare utilization patterns, helping to guide adjustments in trial design.
    - **Incorporating RWE into Adaptive Trials**: The integration of RWE into adaptive trial designs can improve the flexibility and speed of trials, enabling quicker decision-making. For example, if early results show certain

patient groups are responding better to a therapy, the trial design can be adapted to focus on these groups.
- **Examples of Adaptive Trials**: For example, a clinical trial studying a new treatment for cancer might use RWE data on how similar patients have responded to treatments in clinical practice, enabling researchers to identify biomarkers or subgroups that are more likely to benefit from the treatment.

2. **Pragmatic Trials**:
    - **Pragmatic Trials**: These trials are designed to assess the effectiveness of interventions in real-world settings, as opposed to the controlled environments of traditional RCTs. RWE plays a key role in the design of pragmatic trials, as it helps identify the most appropriate outcomes, interventions, and patient populations that reflect real-world practices.
    - **Regulatory Use of Pragmatic Trials**: Regulatory bodies such as the FDA are increasingly looking at pragmatic trial results when evaluating treatments, especially for chronic conditions or complex diseases where real-world application is crucial for understanding the full benefit-risk profile.

3. **Post-Marketing Surveillance**:
    - **Real-World Data for Safety Monitoring**: After a product has been approved, RWE is invaluable in post-marketing surveillance (also known as Phase IV studies), where it helps to track long-term safety, adverse

effects, and adherence in a diverse patient population. This data allows regulatory bodies to monitor for rare adverse events that may not have been apparent in clinical trials.
- **Risk Management Plans**: In some cases, regulatory agencies require ongoing studies based on RWE as part of a risk management plan to ensure continued safety monitoring for drugs, especially those with known risks or for new drug classes.

Case Studies Of Regulatory Approval Based On Rwe

1. **Case Study 1: Use of RWE in Cancer Drugs**:
    - **Example**: The approval of certain oncology drugs has been influenced by RWE, particularly when clinical trial data is insufficient to predict long-term outcomes. For example, the approval of **Kymriah**, a CAR T-cell therapy for certain types of blood cancers, was supported by RWE data showing its effectiveness in a broader population than that which participated in clinical trials.
    - **FDA's Acceptance of RWE**: The FDA acknowledged real-world data from patient registries and observational studies to support the broader use of such therapies.
2. **Case Study 2: Rare Diseases and Orphan Drugs**:
    - **Example**: The approval of **Spinraza** (nusinersen) for Spinal Muscular Atrophy (SMA) was partly based on RWE, as there were very few patients enrolled in the

clinical trials due to the rare nature of the disease. RWE gathered from patients using the drug post-marketing helped confirm its benefit-risk profile.
- **FDA's Support for Rare Diseases**: For orphan drugs, where the patient population is small and traditional clinical trials are not always feasible, RWE can provide valuable evidence to support regulatory approval and ongoing monitoring.

Real-World Evidence For Rare Diseases And Orphan Drugs

1. **Challenges in Rare Disease Research**:
   - Rare diseases present a unique challenge for traditional clinical trials due to the small patient populations. In these cases, it is often difficult to conduct large-scale RCTs. RWE can help overcome these challenges by providing data on disease progression, treatment outcomes, and safety from real-world sources.
   - **Orphan Drug Act**: In the United States, the Orphan Drug Act incentivizes the development of treatments for rare diseases. RWE plays a critical role in this space by providing data on the drug's effects in small patient populations who may not be represented in conventional clinical trials.
2. **Case Example: Duchenne Muscular Dystrophy**:
   - RWE has played a role in the approval of treatments for **Duchenne muscular**

dystrophy (DMD), a rare genetic condition. Due to the difficulty in enrolling large numbers of patients in trials, real-world data has been used to support clinical trial results and provide additional evidence of treatment benefits.

Challenges And Controversies In Rwe Adoption By Regulatory Bodies

1. **Data Quality and Integrity:**
    - **Limitations of RWD**: One of the primary challenges with RWE is ensuring the quality, completeness, and accuracy of real-world data. Unlike controlled clinical trials, RWD may suffer from biases, such as confounding factors, missing data, and incomplete patient records.
    - **Addressing Data Gaps**: Regulatory bodies are concerned about the robustness of RWE, particularly when it is used to inform decisions about approval or label changes. Ensuring proper data validation, standardization, and quality control is essential for gaining regulatory acceptance.
2. **Lack of Standardization:**
    - **Diverse Data Sources**: RWE comes from a variety of sources, including EHRs, insurance claims, and patient registries, which may lack standardization in terms of data collection methods, coding systems, and outcome definitions. This diversity can make it difficult to draw reliable conclusions from RWE alone.

- **Regulatory Hurdles**: Regulatory agencies require rigorous evidence standards, and many of the current frameworks for evaluating RWE are still evolving. Ensuring that RWE meets these high standards can be a complex and time-consuming process.

3. **Resistance to Change**:
    - **Regulatory Reluctance**: Some regulatory agencies may be hesitant to adopt RWE due to concerns about its reliability compared to randomized clinical trials. There is often a lack of experience or formal guidelines for assessing the quality of RWE, leading to resistance or cautious acceptance.
    - **Education and Training**: There is a need for greater education within regulatory bodies about the strengths and limitations of RWE. As more evidence accumulates and frameworks for evaluating RWE are developed, resistance may decrease.

CHAPTER 6: RWE IN HEALTH ECONOMICS AND OUTCOMES RESEARCH

Real-World Evidence (RWE) has emerged as a valuable tool in health economics and outcomes research (HEOR), providing insights into the effectiveness, safety, and overall value of medical interventions in real-world settings.

RWE's ability to reflect actual patient experiences and outcomes in diverse populations makes it essential for understanding the broader impact of healthcare interventions.

The Role Of Rwe In Cost-Effectiveness Analysis

1. **Understanding Cost-Effectiveness Analysis (CEA):**
    - **What is CEA?**: Cost-effectiveness analysis (CEA) is a critical method used in health economics to assess the relative costs and outcomes of different interventions. It helps determine the most efficient allocation of healthcare resources by comparing the cost per unit of health benefit (e.g., quality-adjusted life years, or QALYs) for various treatment options.
    - **Traditional vs. Real-World Data**: While clinical trial data is the gold standard for efficacy, cost-effectiveness assessments based on randomized controlled trials (RCTs) can be limited by their narrow,

controlled environments. RWE enhances CEA by providing data from diverse patient populations, reflecting real-world conditions, comorbidities, and treatment adherence patterns that are often absent in RCTs.

2. **Improved Generalizability**:
    - **Broader Patient Populations**: RWE incorporates data from patients who may have been excluded from clinical trials due to age, comorbid conditions, or other factors. This broader patient base provides a more accurate reflection of the real-world effectiveness of a treatment, making CEA results more generalizable and relevant to diverse healthcare systems.
    - **Diverse Healthcare Settings**: Unlike clinical trials, RWE captures outcomes from a variety of healthcare settings, including primary care, specialist clinics, and hospitals, which may differ significantly in terms of care delivery and patient outcomes. This diversity allows for more accurate modeling of real-world treatment costs and outcomes.

3. **Cost Savings and Real-World Impact**:
    - **Resource Utilization**: RWE can also capture data on healthcare resource utilization, such as hospitalization rates, emergency visits, and medication adherence, providing a more accurate picture of the total cost of care. These insights can help identify cost-saving strategies, optimize treatment pathways, and reduce unnecessary healthcare

expenditures.
- **Long-Term Effects**: RWE can track the long-term effects of treatments, capturing delayed benefits or harms that may not be evident in short-term clinical trials. This extended perspective is essential for modeling the full economic impact of treatments over a patient's lifetime.

Economic Modeling And Cost-Effectiveness Outcomes

1. **Building Economic Models Using RWE**:
    - **Decision-Analytic Models**: Health economists often use decision-analytic models, such as Markov models or discrete event simulation, to simulate the progression of diseases and treatment outcomes over time. These models typically incorporate both clinical trial data and RWE to estimate long-term costs and health outcomes.
    - **Real-World Data in Economic Models**: The integration of RWE into these models enhances their external validity. RWE allows for more realistic assumptions regarding patient characteristics, disease progression, treatment adherence, and outcomes, which can improve the accuracy and applicability of cost-effectiveness models.
2. **Cost-Effectiveness Outcomes**:

- **Incremental Cost-Effectiveness Ratio (ICER)**: One of the primary metrics used in CEA is the incremental cost-effectiveness ratio (ICER), which compares the additional cost of a treatment to its additional health benefit, typically measured in QALYs. RWE can provide more accurate estimates of ICER by using data on real-world costs and health outcomes.
- **Real-World Data for Sensitivity Analysis**: Sensitivity analysis is often performed in economic models to assess the robustness of the results under varying assumptions. RWE provides the necessary data to conduct these analyses in a more realistic context, testing how changes in factors such as patient demographics, treatment adherence, and comorbidities impact cost-effectiveness.

Patient-Reported Outcomes (Pros) And Quality Of Life (Qol) Assessments

1. **Patient-Reported Outcomes (PROs):**
    - **Defining PROs**: PROs are direct reports from patients about their health status without interpretation by healthcare professionals. PROs typically include measures of symptoms, functional status, treatment satisfaction, and emotional well-being. These measures are crucial for understanding how patients perceive their health and the impact of treatments on their day-to-day lives.
    - **Real-World Applications**: RWE often

includes PROs, providing a more comprehensive view of treatment effectiveness. In clinical trials, PROs may be limited by strict inclusion criteria or controlled settings. In contrast, real-world data can capture a broader spectrum of patient experiences, enabling the evaluation of treatment outcomes in diverse populations with varying levels of disease severity.

2. **Quality of Life (QoL) Assessments**:
   - **Understanding QoL**: QoL assessments are a vital component of health outcomes research, focusing on the patient's overall well-being, including physical, mental, and social functioning. QoL metrics are often used in conjunction with PROs to assess the broader impact of medical interventions on a patient's life.
   - **Impact of RWE on QoL Studies**: RWE provides valuable insights into QoL by capturing data from routine clinical care, where patients may face real-life challenges not represented in controlled trials. By evaluating QoL in real-world settings, RWE can help identify the long-term effects of treatments on patients' daily lives and contribute to understanding the full benefits of interventions.

Value-Based Healthcare And Its Relation To Rwe

1. **The Concept of Value-Based Healthcare**:
   - **Defining Value-Based Healthcare**: Value-

based healthcare focuses on improving patient outcomes while controlling costs. It shifts the emphasis from the volume of services provided to the value created by healthcare interventions. The value of care is typically measured by health outcomes relative to costs, making it highly relevant to economic evaluations in healthcare.

- **RWE's Role in Value Assessment**: RWE plays a crucial role in the transition to value-based healthcare by providing evidence of treatment effectiveness, safety, and costs in real-world settings. Unlike traditional models that prioritize clinical efficacy in controlled trials, value-based models emphasize outcomes that matter most to patients, such as quality of life, symptom relief, and functional improvement.

2. **Real-World Value Demonstration**:

    - **Proving Value Beyond Efficacy**: RWE can help demonstrate the value of treatments in real-world contexts, considering factors such as patient adherence, access to care, and broader health outcomes. This is particularly important for therapies that provide benefits beyond the traditional clinical endpoints used in trials.

    - **Patient-Centered Measures**: RWE incorporates a range of patient-centered outcomes, including PROs and QoL metrics, which are essential for evaluating the true value of interventions from the patient's perspective. This helps ensure that value-based healthcare models reflect what matters most to patients, including their ability to lead fulfilling lives with manageable health conditions.

Case Studies Of Rwe In Pricing And Reimbursement Decisions

1. **Case Study 1: Pricing of Hepatitis C Medications**:
   - **Background**: The introduction of direct-acting antiviral (DAA) medications for hepatitis C has revolutionized treatment, offering high cure rates. However, the high cost of these therapies posed a challenge for healthcare systems.
   - **Use of RWE**: RWE was used to demonstrate the long-term benefits of these medications, such as reduced healthcare costs due to decreased liver transplants and lower rates of liver cancer. By integrating RWE into pricing negotiations, manufacturers were able to justify the high initial costs of the drugs by showing their long-term cost-effectiveness.
   - **Reimbursement Decisions**: Healthcare payers and insurers incorporated RWE into their reimbursement decisions, agreeing to cover these treatments based on the demonstrated long-term savings, improving access to these life-saving therapies.
2. **Case Study 2: Oncology Drug Pricing and Value Assessment**:

- **Background**: The pricing of oncology drugs, particularly those for metastatic cancer, has been a point of contention due to their high costs relative to the clinical benefits demonstrated in trials. However, RWE has been used to supplement trial data and justify pricing decisions.
- **Use of RWE**: RWE has provided evidence of how oncology treatments perform in a broader patient population, including those with comorbidities or varying cancer stages. Additionally, data on real-world survival rates and symptom improvement has supported the justification for pricing and reimbursement decisions.
- **Outcome**: Payers have increasingly considered RWE in their value-based assessments, ensuring that the pricing of oncology drugs reflects both clinical outcomes and patient quality of life in real-world settings.

CHAPTER 7: REAL-WORLD EVIDENCE IN DRUG DEVELOPMENT AND POST-MARKET SURVEILLANCE

Real-World Evidence (RWE) has transformed drug development and post-market surveillance by complementing traditional clinical trials with data that reflects the actual use of medications in broader patient populations.

Rwe In The Preclinical And Clinical Phases Of Drug Development

1. **Role of RWE in Early Drug Development**:
    - **Identifying Unmet Medical Needs**: In the early stages of drug development, RWE can help identify patient populations with unmet medical needs. Data from patient registries, electronic health records (EHRs), and other sources can shed light on disease prevalence, treatment gaps, and potential candidates for novel therapies. RWE allows for a better understanding of disease heterogeneity, helping pharmaceutical companies design clinical trials that target the most relevant populations.
    - **Accelerating Development with RWE**: For certain conditions, RWE can accelerate the

preclinical phase by providing insights into the disease mechanism, progression, and prior treatment outcomes. In some cases, RWE might be used to support adaptive trial designs, which allow for modifications to ongoing trials based on real-time data analysis.

2. **Supporting Phase I and II Clinical Trials with RWE:**
    - **Patient Recruitment and Inclusion Criteria**: Traditional clinical trials often have strict inclusion and exclusion criteria, which can limit the generalizability of the results. RWE helps in identifying broader, more diverse patient populations who could benefit from experimental treatments. By analyzing real-world data from clinical registries and health databases, researchers can refine patient recruitment strategies and select participants who more accurately represent the target population.
    - **Patient Characteristics and Treatment Pathways**: RWE can be used to identify common comorbidities, concurrent treatments, and disease progression patterns in patients, allowing drug developers to account for these factors in clinical trial design. This leads to better-informed, more realistic trials that reflect actual patient experiences, improving the potential for real-world success once the drug is marketed.
3. **Incorporating RWE into Phase III Trials:**
    - **Optimizing Trial Design**: While Phase III clinical trials remain the gold standard

for establishing drug efficacy, incorporating RWE can enhance these trials by providing context for the expected outcomes. For example, data from EHRs or observational studies can inform the design of more robust control groups and endpoints. By integrating real-world evidence, researchers can ensure the trial's findings are more aligned with how a drug will perform in the broader population.

- **Predicting Real-World Efficacy**: Using RWE, researchers can model expected outcomes in the general population based on pre-existing patient data. This can provide early insights into how the drug may perform after approval, helping to inform the design of subsequent trials and regulatory submissions.

Post-Market Surveillance And Monitoring Of Adverse Events (Pharmacovigilance)

1. **Pharmacovigilance and RWE:**
    - **Role of RWE in Safety Monitoring**: After a drug is approved and released into the market, ongoing surveillance is essential to detect adverse events (AEs) and assess the drug's safety profile over time. Traditional post-market surveillance relies on spontaneous reporting systems, such as the FDA's Adverse Event Reporting System (FAERS) or the EMA's EudraVigilance. However, these systems are limited by underreporting and reporting biases.

- **Enhancing Safety Monitoring with RWE:** RWE enhances pharmacovigilance by incorporating data from various sources, such as insurance claims, electronic health records, and patient registries. By analyzing large-scale, real-world data sets, researchers can identify previously unreported or rare side effects, especially those that may not have emerged in clinical trials due to their limited sample size and controlled environments.

2. **Identifying Adverse Drug Reactions (ADRs):**
    - **Long-Term Safety:** While clinical trials typically monitor patients for a few months to a few years, RWE allows for the continuous monitoring of a drug's safety profile over a longer period. This includes tracking late-onset adverse drug reactions (ADRs), which may not be evident in the clinical trial phase.
    - **Uncommon and Rare Side Effects:** Some adverse effects are so rare that they would be unlikely to appear in the controlled environment of a clinical trial. With RWE, large datasets can be leveraged to detect these rare events once the drug is widely available. For example, patients with comorbidities or those on multiple medications can reveal side effects that wouldn't be captured in clinical trials involving more homogenous patient groups.

3. **Signal Detection and Risk Management:**
    - **Signal Detection:** RWE is instrumental in signal detection—identifying potential

safety concerns that require further investigation. Machine learning and advanced statistical techniques can analyze vast amounts of real-world data to detect unusual patterns or spikes in adverse events, allowing regulatory bodies to act quickly to mitigate risks.
- **Risk Management**: Post-market surveillance often includes risk management strategies, such as risk communication plans and risk minimization strategies (e.g., restricted distribution). By continuously monitoring real-world data, manufacturers can adjust their risk management strategies in response to emerging safety concerns.

Identifying Long-Term Outcomes And Rare Side Effects

1. **Long-Term Efficacy and Safety**:
    - **RWE for Long-Term Outcomes**: While clinical trials may assess the short- and medium-term outcomes of a drug, RWE is invaluable in understanding its long-term effects. For chronic conditions, data from long-term cohort studies, registries, and insurance claims can be used to assess the sustained efficacy of treatments and any delayed adverse effects.
    - **Chronic Disease Management**: RWE provides insights into how medications affect patients over the course of years, particularly in chronic diseases where the benefits and risks of treatment evolve over

time. For instance, in cardiovascular or diabetes treatment, RWE can reveal the long-term impact of medications on outcomes like heart attack rates, hospitalizations, and life expectancy.

2. **Rare Adverse Events:**
    - **Capturing Rare Side Effects**: Clinical trials typically have a limited sample size, which means that rare adverse events may not be detected during pre-market testing. RWE, however, can identify these side effects by analyzing data from large, diverse patient populations once a drug is on the market.
    - **Example**: The detection of rare adverse effects, such as drug-induced liver injury, is one example of how RWE has contributed to drug safety monitoring after market approval. By monitoring real-world health records, physicians, and regulators can quickly spot such issues and respond accordingly.

Real-World Data In Comparative Effectiveness Research

1. **Comparative Effectiveness Research (CER):**
    - **What is CER?**: Comparative effectiveness research compares the outcomes, risks, and benefits of different treatment options to determine which works best for a particular patient population. This is particularly valuable when multiple treatment options are available for the same condition, as it helps guide healthcare providers in selecting

the most effective and safe treatments.
- **RWE in CER**: Unlike randomized controlled trials (RCTs), which are often limited by strict inclusion criteria, RWE in CER incorporates data from broader, more diverse patient populations. It helps to evaluate treatments under typical clinical conditions, accounting for factors such as comorbidities, polypharmacy, and adherence issues that may not be present in controlled trials.

2. **Assessing Real-World Effectiveness**:
   - **Effectiveness in Real-World Settings**: While RCTs measure the efficacy of a treatment in controlled conditions, RWE helps assess how well the treatment works when deployed in the broader population. This includes evaluating the treatment's effectiveness in different subpopulations, such as elderly patients, pregnant women, or those with multiple comorbidities.

The Use Of Rwe To Inform Drug Labeling And Treatment Guidelines

1. **Influencing Drug Labeling**:
   - **Expanding Drug Labels**: Regulatory agencies like the FDA and EMA can use RWE to update drug labels with new indications, dosing recommendations, or safety warnings based on real-world data. For example, if real-world evidence shows that a drug is effective for a broader patient population than originally studied in clinical

trials, this can lead to label expansions.
- **Safety Warnings**: RWE can also inform the inclusion of new safety warnings on drug labels if post-market surveillance reveals previously unreported adverse events. The ability to quickly update drug labels with new safety information is crucial for protecting patient health.

2. **Guideline Development**:
   - **Guideline Recommendations**: Treatment guidelines are often based on evidence from randomized controlled trials. However, as RWE grows in importance, it increasingly informs clinical practice guidelines by providing a more comprehensive view of how drugs perform in the real world. RWE can help shape guidelines for conditions where treatment options are varied and outcomes are influenced by factors not addressed in RCTs.
   - **Example**: In oncology, RWE has been used to inform guidelines for the use of certain immunotherapies and targeted therapies, especially when clinical trial data is limited or lacks generalizability to specific patient subgroups.

CHAPTER 8: CHALLENGES AND LIMITATIONS OF REAL-WORLD EVIDENCE

While Real-World Evidence (RWE) has revolutionized clinical research by providing insights into the effectiveness, safety, and outcomes of treatments in actual clinical practice, its application is not without challenges.

RWE relies heavily on observational data, which introduces several limitations.

1. Data Quality And Completeness Issues In Real-World Data (Rwd)

Real-World Data (RWD) is often collected from diverse and non-standardized sources, such as Electronic Health Records (EHRs), insurance claims, patient registries, and wearable devices. While these data sources offer valuable insights, they are prone to several issues that can compromise their quality and completeness.

- **Inconsistent Data Collection**: One of the primary challenges in RWD is the inconsistency in data collection methods across different sources. For example, EHRs may include different types of information depending on the healthcare system or hospital, leading to variations in the quality and comprehensiveness of data.
- **Missing Data**: Data gaps are common in RWD,

whether due to patient non-compliance, incomplete documentation, or healthcare providers not entering all relevant information. Missing data can skew results and limit the conclusions that can be drawn from a study.

- **Data Standardization**: RWD often comes from multiple systems with varying formats, codes, and terminologies. Lack of standardization in data entry practices can make it difficult to harmonize datasets for analysis. Data preprocessing and transformation are essential steps, but they can be time-consuming and may introduce errors if not handled carefully.

Solution: One potential solution is the use of data standardization frameworks (such as the Common Data Model for clinical research), which help in harmonizing data formats across different sources and improving data comparability.

2. Selection Bias and Confounding Factors

Unlike randomized controlled trials (RCTs), where patients are randomly assigned to treatment and control groups, RWE studies are typically observational in nature, meaning that there is no randomization. This introduces the possibility of selection bias and confounding factors that can distort the findings.

- **Selection Bias**: In observational studies, the treatment assignment is not randomized, so certain groups of patients may be more likely to receive a specific treatment due to factors such as disease severity, age, comorbidities, or socio-economic status. This leads to selection bias, where the treatment group may not be representative of the general population, affecting the generalizability of the results.
- **Confounding**: Confounding occurs when an external variable is associated with both the treatment and

the outcome, leading to a spurious relationship between them. For example, patients who receive a particular drug may be more likely to have better access to healthcare or healthier lifestyles, which could contribute to better outcomes independently of the treatment.

Solution: Statistical techniques such as propensity score matching, regression models, and inverse probability weighting can be used to adjust for selection bias and confounding. However, these methods have limitations and may not fully eliminate the effects of bias.

3. Ethical Challenges In Real-World Data Collection And Usage

The collection and use of RWD in clinical research raise several ethical issues related to privacy, informed consent, and the potential for misuse of sensitive data.

- **Privacy and Data Protection**: One of the most significant ethical concerns in RWD research is patient privacy. Data sources such as EHRs, insurance claims, and social media often contain sensitive personal information. If this data is not anonymized or de-identified properly, it could lead to privacy violations or breaches of confidentiality.
- **Informed Consent**: Unlike clinical trials, where patients provide explicit informed consent to participate, RWE studies often use existing datasets without direct patient involvement. This raises concerns about whether patients are adequately informed about how their data will be used, especially if the data was collected for purposes other than

research.
- **Data Misuse**: There is also a risk that RWD could be used for purposes other than originally intended, such as marketing or policy decisions, without proper oversight. This could undermine patient trust in healthcare systems and research initiatives.

Solution: Strong ethical guidelines and regulatory frameworks, such as the General Data Protection Regulation (GDPR) in Europe and the Health Insurance Portability and Accountability Act (HIPAA) in the United States, can help mitigate these concerns.

Additionally, using secure data storage methods, ensuring patient consent where possible, and maintaining transparency in research practices are essential to preserving ethical standards.

4. Issues Related To The Generalizability Of Real-World Evidence

One of the core advantages of RWE is its ability to reflect outcomes in real-world settings, but this can also be a limitation when it comes to generalizability. Real-world populations are often heterogeneous, and RWE studies may struggle to provide findings that are applicable to all groups.

- **Patient Heterogeneity**: RWE studies often include patients with diverse demographics, comorbid conditions, and varying treatment histories. While this diversity provides a more comprehensive view of how treatments perform in practice, it also means that the results may not be easily generalizable to specific subgroups or settings.
- **Variation in Healthcare Practices**: Different healthcare

systems and practices (e.g., public vs. private healthcare, variations in physician practices) can lead to inconsistent treatment protocols and outcomes. This variability can limit the ability to draw universal conclusions from RWE studies.

- **External Validity**: Even though RWE studies can offer insights into treatment outcomes under real-world conditions, the findings might not always be transferable to other populations or settings, especially in the case of rare diseases or highly specific subpopulations.

Solution: To improve generalizability, researchers can conduct subgroup analyses to understand how different populations respond to treatments. Additionally, cross-validation using data from multiple, diverse sources can help ensure that the findings are more widely applicable.

5. Overcoming The Limitations Of Observational Studies In Rwe

Since RWE relies heavily on observational data, it inherits many of the limitations associated with this type of research design. However, various strategies can be employed to mitigate these limitations and enhance the reliability of findings.

- **Use of Advanced Statistical Methods**: Techniques such as propensity score matching, regression adjustment, and instrumental variable analysis can help control for confounders and biases in observational data. These methods aim to replicate the conditions of a randomized controlled trial as much as possible, providing more robust estimates of treatment effects.
- **Sensitivity Analysis**: Sensitivity analyses can be used to test the robustness of the results to different

assumptions or methods of analysis. This helps researchers identify whether their findings hold under varying conditions or if they are driven by specific methodological choices.

- **Longitudinal Data Collection**: While observational studies often have limitations in terms of causality, longitudinal data collection (tracking patients over time) can help establish temporal relationships between exposure and outcomes, providing stronger evidence for causal inference.
- **Hybrid Study Designs**: Hybrid study designs, which combine RWE with elements of randomized controlled trials, are gaining traction. These designs may include randomized components within observational studies, helping to overcome some of the biases inherent in purely observational approaches.

Solution: By combining rigorous statistical methods, well-designed study protocols, and hybrid approaches, researchers can mitigate the limitations of observational studies and enhance the credibility and accuracy of RWE findings.

CHAPTER 9: THE FUTURE OF REAL-WORLD EVIDENCE

Real-World Evidence (RWE) has already made a significant impact on clinical research, regulatory decision-making, and healthcare policy.

As technological advancements continue to evolve, the future of RWE promises to enhance the scope, precision, and real-time applicability of healthcare research.

1. Innovations In Rwe Methodology: Big Data, Ai, And Machine Learning

The use of **big data**, **artificial intelligence (AI)**, and **machine learning** in RWE studies is rapidly advancing and transforming how clinical research is conducted. These technologies offer a vast array of opportunities to improve data analysis, uncover new insights, and predict healthcare outcomes with greater accuracy and efficiency.

- **Big Data Integration**: As healthcare data sources continue to grow in both volume and diversity (including EHRs, wearables, genomics, social media, and more), big data technologies are essential for processing, analyzing, and making sense of this wealth of information. The integration of large datasets from multiple sources enables researchers to better understand population health trends and treatment effectiveness across different demographics.
- **Artificial Intelligence (AI) and Machine Learning**:

AI and machine learning algorithms are increasingly being used to analyze complex RWD. These algorithms can identify patterns and relationships in data that might not be apparent through traditional statistical methods. AI can also help automate processes such as data cleaning, anomaly detection, and predictive modeling, enhancing the efficiency of RWE studies. Furthermore, machine learning techniques, such as supervised learning and deep learning, are being employed to build predictive models for patient outcomes, optimize treatment plans, and identify previously unknown side effects of drugs.

- **Natural Language Processing (NLP)**: NLP is another AI-based technology that can be leveraged in RWE research. It allows for the extraction of valuable insights from unstructured data sources, such as clinical notes, medical literature, and patient-reported outcomes. NLP can help transform these textual data into usable information, enabling more comprehensive analyses and insights.

The Future: The future of RWE will see a more seamless integration of big data, AI, and machine learning, leading to faster and more accurate predictions of treatment outcomes, healthcare trends, and patient behavior. Additionally, AI-powered real-time monitoring systems could revolutionize the way adverse events and patient outcomes are tracked.

2. Real-Time Data Collection And Patient Monitoring Technologies

The future of RWE will also be heavily shaped by advancements in **real-time data collection** and **patient monitoring technologies**. As more patients engage with digital health tools, the opportunity for researchers to collect continuous, real-time data on patient health and treatment response is becoming a reality.

- **Wearable Devices**: Devices such as smartwatches, fitness trackers, and other wearables are increasingly being used to monitor vital signs, physical activity, and other health metrics. These devices provide continuous, real-time data that can be integrated into RWE studies. By using wearables to track patients' health status outside of traditional healthcare settings, researchers can gain deeper insights into how treatments perform in real-world conditions.
- **Mobile Health Apps (mHealth)**: Mobile health apps are playing an increasingly important role in patient monitoring. These apps can track symptoms, treatment adherence, medication usage, and other health-related data, providing a rich source of real-world information. Many mHealth apps are now integrated with healthcare systems, allowing for direct reporting of patient data to healthcare providers and researchers.
- **Remote Patient Monitoring (RPM)**: RPM technologies enable healthcare providers to monitor patients outside of the clinical setting, reducing the need for in-person visits and allowing for the continuous collection of health data. This is particularly important for chronic disease management and for populations that may have difficulty accessing traditional healthcare facilities.

The Future: Real-time data collection technologies will continue to evolve, providing a more comprehensive and accurate picture of patient health. The integration of real-time monitoring into clinical trials and RWE studies will enable researchers to capture data on adverse events, treatment adherence, and long-term outcomes in a much more efficient and timely manner.

This will facilitate more accurate decision-making and timely interventions.

3. The Role Of Patient-Centric Approaches In Rwe

A growing focus on **patient-centered research** is increasingly influencing the design and execution of RWE studies. Patient engagement and empowerment are essential for improving the quality and applicability of real-world evidence.

In this context, technologies such as **mobile health apps, patient registries**, and **social media** are becoming powerful tools for incorporating patient perspectives into RWE research.

- **Patient Engagement**: Involving patients in the design and execution of RWE studies can enhance the relevance and applicability of research findings. Patients can provide valuable insights into their treatment experiences, preferences, and quality of life, which can help tailor treatments and improve outcomes. Patient engagement platforms and digital tools that facilitate communication between patients and researchers will continue to evolve, allowing for more collaborative and patient-centered studies.
- **Patient-Reported Outcomes (PROs)**: PROs are increasingly recognized as critical components of RWE. These self-reported measures, collected through surveys or digital tools, capture the patient's perspective on their health status, symptoms, and quality of life. Incorporating PROs into RWE studies enables researchers to evaluate treatments not just in terms of clinical endpoints but also from the viewpoint of patients themselves.
- **Mobile Health Apps and Social Media**: These technologies provide new avenues for engaging with

patients and collecting real-world data. Social media platforms can serve as informal channels for patient feedback, while mobile apps facilitate ongoing patient engagement and data collection, allowing researchers to follow patients over long periods of time.

The Future: As patient-centered approaches become more widespread, future RWE studies will increasingly prioritize patient involvement and use innovative technologies to gather insights that reflect real-world patient experiences. These approaches will help tailor treatments to individual needs and improve patient outcomes.

4. Policy And Regulatory Changes Supporting The Integration Of Rwe

Regulatory bodies, such as the **FDA**, **EMA**, and **Health Canada**, are increasingly acknowledging the value of Real-World Evidence in shaping healthcare decisions. As these organizations recognize the potential of RWE, they are adapting their policies to support the integration of real-world data into clinical research and regulatory processes.

- **Regulatory Guidelines**: The FDA and other regulatory agencies have issued guidelines that allow RWE to be used in drug approval processes, especially for post-marketing surveillance and rare disease treatments. These agencies are working to develop frameworks for the appropriate use of RWE in regulatory submissions, ensuring that it complements traditional clinical trial data while maintaining rigorous scientific standards.
- **Adaptive Clinical Trial Designs**: The integration of RWE into adaptive clinical trials is a significant development. These trials are designed to be more flexible, incorporating real-world data to modify

aspects of the study (e.g., dosage, treatment protocol) based on emerging evidence. This allows for quicker adjustments and a more responsive approach to patient care.

- **Accelerated Approvals for Rare Diseases**: RWE has proven invaluable in advancing treatments for rare diseases and orphan drugs, where clinical trial data may be scarce due to small patient populations. Regulatory bodies are increasingly using RWE to accelerate approval processes for these treatments, shortening the time it takes for patients to access life-saving therapies.

The Future: Ongoing changes in regulatory frameworks will likely further integrate RWE into the clinical development process, providing more robust evidence for regulatory submissions and supporting the approval of innovative treatments. Policy reforms will continue to adapt to the growing importance of real-world data in improving healthcare outcomes.

5. The Evolving Role Of Rwe In Precision Medicine And Personalized Healthcare

As healthcare moves toward more **personalized treatment** approaches, the role of Real-World Evidence in **precision medicine** will become even more crucial. Precision medicine tailors medical treatment to the individual characteristics of each patient, such as their genetic makeup, lifestyle, and environmental factors.

- **Genomic Data Integration**: The integration of genomic data with real-world health data will allow for more precise predictions about treatment responses. By understanding how genetic variations affect drug metabolism and treatment outcomes, researchers can use RWE to identify the most effective therapies for

different genetic subgroups.
- **Biomarker Discovery and Validation**: RWE can be used to identify and validate biomarkers that predict treatment response, disease progression, and other key clinical outcomes. The availability of RWD from diverse patient populations allows for the identification of new biomarkers that may not have been discovered through traditional clinical trials.
- **Personalized Treatment Plans**: With the help of RWE, healthcare providers will be able to create more personalized treatment plans based on the individual characteristics of patients. This will improve the accuracy of diagnosis, optimize treatment regimens, and enhance patient outcomes.

The Future: The future of RWE in *precision medicine* will see increasingly sophisticated integration of genetic, environmental, and lifestyle data, allowing for truly personalized healthcare. This will lead to more effective treatments, fewer side effects, and improved patient satisfaction as healthcare becomes more tailored to individual needs.

CHAPTER 10: CASE STUDIES IN REAL-WORLD EVIDENCE APPLICATIONS

Case Study 1: Using Rwe To Assess The Effectiveness Of A Newly Approved Drug

Background:
After a new drug receives regulatory approval, post-marketing surveillance is crucial to assess its effectiveness and safety in the general population, beyond the controlled settings of clinical trials. Real-World Evidence offers a powerful tool for this type of post-marketing evaluation.

Application:
In this case study, a new treatment for chronic pain (e.g., a non-opioid pain management drug) was approved by the FDA based on results from randomized controlled trials (RCTs). However, the drug's use in the broader, real-world population raised concerns about its long-term effectiveness and safety, as RCTs often include a select population that may not fully represent the diversity of patients who will ultimately use the drug.

RWE was collected from **electronic health records (EHRs)**, **claims data**, and **patient registries**. Researchers conducted an observational study using these data sources to evaluate how the drug performed across different patient subgroups, including those with comorbidities, different age groups, and those on polypharmacy.

Findings:
The RWE study revealed that the drug was generally effective for the majority of patients but had a slightly reduced efficacy in older patients and those with specific pre-existing conditions, such as kidney disease. Additionally, safety signals were identified regarding potential interactions with certain commonly prescribed medications, leading to recommendations for revised usage guidelines.

Impact:
This RWE study helped healthcare providers better understand the drug's real-world performance and led to adjustments in its prescribing information, including dosage recommendations and safety warnings. This case highlights the importance of using RWE to monitor long-term outcomes and refine treatment guidelines after regulatory approval.

Case Study 2: Post-Market Surveillance And Safety Monitoring Of Vaccines

Background:
Vaccines undergo rigorous clinical trials to assess their safety and efficacy. However, post-market surveillance is necessary to monitor their safety in the general population, particularly for detecting rare adverse events that may not be apparent during pre-approval clinical trials due to sample size limitations.

Application:
A new vaccine for a respiratory virus was launched globally, and post-marketing surveillance was established to track adverse events using RWD sources like national immunization registries, hospital databases, and spontaneous reporting systems such as the **Vaccine Adverse Event Reporting System (VAERS)**.

An RWE study was initiated to monitor adverse events and identify any emerging safety concerns that might not have been detected in the clinical trials. Data from multiple countries, including electronic medical records, claims data, and direct patient-reported outcomes, were integrated into a global RWE platform.

Findings:
RWE monitoring revealed a very low incidence of an uncommon adverse event: a specific type of neurological disorder. While the absolute risk was small, the real-world data helped identify specific risk factors, such as age, genetic predispositions, and previous medical history, that made some patients more susceptible to the adverse event.

Impact:
As a result, the vaccine's labeling was updated to include a specific warning for the identified risk factors. Additionally, public health messaging was adapted to ensure informed decision-making by healthcare providers and patients. This case demonstrates how RWE plays a crucial role in ongoing safety monitoring and the identification of previously unrecognized risks in post-marketing surveillance.

Case Study 3: Real-World Data Supporting Health Insurance Reimbursement Decisions

Background:
Health insurance companies often rely on clinical trial data to make reimbursement decisions. However, clinical trial data can sometimes be insufficient to determine how well a treatment works in everyday clinical practice, especially when considering diverse populations with varying comorbidities.

Application:
A new biologic treatment for **rheumatoid arthritis** was approved based on clinical trials but faced challenges in demonstrating its cost-effectiveness and real-world benefits for broad patient populations. Insurers were hesitant to approve full reimbursement without evidence of the drug's effectiveness and cost relative to other treatment options in routine clinical practice.

An RWE study was conducted using claims data, patient registries, and observational cohort studies to compare the effectiveness and cost-effectiveness of the biologic against other existing treatments for rheumatoid arthritis in real-world settings. The analysis focused on metrics such as patient adherence, hospitalizations, and the impact on quality of life.

Findings:
The RWE study demonstrated that the biologic significantly reduced hospital admissions and long-term disability in real-world patients, leading to lower overall healthcare costs due to fewer complications. It also provided evidence of improved patient-reported outcomes and long-term disease control in diverse patient populations, including those with multiple comorbidities.

Impact:
Armed with this evidence, the health insurance company decided to approve reimbursement for the biologic at a reduced cost based on its proven cost-effectiveness in real-world settings. This case highlights how RWE can bridge the gap between clinical trial data and real-world healthcare needs, providing decision-makers with the evidence necessary to make informed reimbursement decisions.

Case Study 4: Rwe In Chronic Disease Management And Prevention Strategies

Background:
Chronic diseases such as **diabetes**, **hypertension**, and **obesity** are major drivers of healthcare costs and morbidity. Prevention and management strategies are often guided by clinical trial evidence, but these strategies may not fully address the complexities of real-world patient populations, who often have comorbid conditions and diverse socio-economic backgrounds.

Application:
An initiative to improve **chronic disease management** through a community-based intervention program used RWE to evaluate the effectiveness of various management strategies. The program utilized a combination of patient-reported outcomes, medical claims data, and health assessments from patients participating in a community health program.

The study aimed to assess the effectiveness of **lifestyle interventions** (such as diet and exercise) versus **pharmacologic treatments** for controlling blood pressure and blood sugar levels in diverse, real-world populations. Data from electronic health records were analyzed to compare the long-term outcomes of these interventions in managing chronic disease.

Findings:
The RWE study found that while pharmacologic treatments were effective for short-term control of symptoms, lifestyle interventions had a more sustained positive impact on long-term outcomes such as weight loss, blood pressure, and blood sugar control. Additionally, the data indicated that combining lifestyle interventions with pharmacological treatment improved patient outcomes more than either intervention alone.

Impact:
These findings were used to advocate for policy changes, recommending increased support for lifestyle-based interventions in chronic disease management programs. This case underscores the importance of RWE in shaping effective, patient-centered strategies for chronic disease management and prevention.

Case Study 5: Using Rwe To Assess Treatment Patterns And Outcomes In Rare Diseases

Background:
Rare diseases often lack the robust clinical trial data needed to develop comprehensive treatment guidelines. Given the small number of patients, clinical trials can be difficult to conduct. RWE offers an alternative means of understanding disease progression and treatment outcomes in these populations.

Application:
A treatment for **rare genetic disorder X** was approved based on limited clinical trial data, but clinicians needed more information about the drug's effectiveness in treating the disease in real-world settings. An RWE study was initiated to assess treatment patterns and long-term outcomes using data from national disease registries, EHRs, and patient surveys.

The study tracked patients with **genetic disorder X** who were treated with the new drug, comparing outcomes such as symptom progression, hospitalizations, and survival rates with patients who had not received the treatment. Researchers also gathered data on the management of co-occurring conditions and patient quality of life.

Findings:
The study showed that the new treatment improved both clinical outcomes (such as reduced disease progression) and patient-reported quality of life. However, it also revealed that access to the treatment was limited by socio-economic factors, leading to disparities in treatment outcomes. These insights were critical for understanding how the treatment works in a real-world setting.

Impact:
The findings contributed to the development of more targeted treatment guidelines for rare disease X and helped inform reimbursement policies. Additionally, the study highlighted the need for better access to therapies for underserved populations. This case illustrates the power of RWE in filling the gaps in knowledge for rare diseases, where traditional clinical trials are often not feasible.

Case Study 6: Rwe In Cardiovascular Disease Management

Background:
Cardiovascular diseases (CVD) are leading causes of morbidity and mortality worldwide. Clinical trials provide essential data for cardiovascular treatments, but their findings may not always reflect the complexities of real-world patient populations, which often include individuals with multiple comorbidities or high-risk profiles.

Application:
A study was designed to evaluate the effectiveness of a new **antiplatelet therapy** for patients with **acute coronary syndrome (ACS)** in real-world clinical settings. The therapy had been approved based on clinical trials, but its real-world performance, especially in older adults and those with comorbid conditions like

diabetes or hypertension, needed further exploration.

RWE was collected from a large **insurance claims database** and **EHRs** across multiple hospitals. The data captured patient demographics, comorbidities, treatment regimens, and long-term outcomes like hospital readmission rates, adverse events, and mortality.

Findings:
The RWE analysis showed that the antiplatelet therapy was effective in reducing **heart attack recurrence** and hospital readmissions. However, patients with poorly controlled diabetes or advanced kidney disease had a higher incidence of adverse events. Moreover, patients receiving the therapy in combination with statins showed improved long-term outcomes compared to those on monotherapy.

Impact:
These findings led to recommendations for **personalized treatment regimens**, where the new antiplatelet therapy was advised alongside statins for patients with diabetes and cardiovascular disease. This case illustrates how RWE can guide tailored treatment approaches in chronic disease management.

Case Study 7: Rwe In Pediatric Asthma Management

Background:
Asthma is a common chronic condition in children, and treatment guidelines often rely on clinical trial data. However, the variability in asthma severity and triggers across the pediatric

population means that real-world data is crucial to better understand how treatments perform in daily practice.

Application:
A pharmaceutical company sought to assess the real-world effectiveness of a new inhaled corticosteroid (ICS) for controlling asthma in children. Although the drug was FDA-approved based on clinical trials, there were concerns about adherence and its effectiveness across diverse pediatric populations, including those with concurrent conditions such as **allergic rhinitis** or **eczema**.

An RWE study was designed using **patient registries**, **EHRs**, and data from **mobile health apps** tracking inhaler use, symptom diaries, and healthcare utilization (e.g., emergency visits and hospitalizations). The study aimed to assess medication adherence, symptom control, and healthcare outcomes across a large sample of children in community-based practices.

Findings:
The study found that children with asthma who consistently used the ICS showed a significant reduction in emergency room visits and hospitalization rates. However, adherence was a major issue, with many children failing to take the medication as prescribed. The effectiveness of the ICS was enhanced when paired with educational interventions that encouraged medication adherence.

Impact:
The RWE study led to the development of **adherence support programs**, including mobile reminders and educational campaigns for parents and children. The results highlighted the importance of **patient education** and **regular follow-up** to improve asthma management, particularly in the pediatric population.

Case Study 8: Rwe In Assessing The Impact Of Telemedicine For Mental Health Treatment

Background:
Telemedicine has grown in popularity for providing mental health services, especially in underserved or rural areas. However, its effectiveness compared to traditional in-person therapy needed further investigation, especially regarding long-term outcomes such as patient satisfaction, treatment efficacy, and engagement.

Application:
A large-scale RWE study was conducted to evaluate the effectiveness of **telepsychiatry** for treating **depression** and **anxiety disorders** in adults. Patients were randomly assigned to either telemedicine sessions or traditional face-to-face therapy sessions. Data was collected from **EHRs**, **patient surveys**, and **telemedicine platform records** to assess clinical outcomes (e.g., symptom reduction) and patient satisfaction.

Findings:
The study revealed that telepsychiatry was equally effective as in-person therapy in reducing symptoms of depression and anxiety. Patients in both groups showed similar improvements in clinical scales (e.g., **PHQ-9** for depression). However, patients who participated in telepsychiatry were more likely to attend sessions due to the convenience of virtual appointments. Satisfaction scores were slightly higher among telemedicine patients, with many citing the flexibility of virtual sessions as a key benefit.

Impact:
Based on these findings, healthcare providers and insurers began to expand access to telepsychiatry services, particularly in rural

and underserved regions. The RWE study provided evidence supporting the **long-term feasibility** of telemedicine in mental health care, influencing insurance reimbursement policies and integration into standard mental health practices.

Case Study 9: Rwe In Evaluating Diabetes Management Technologies

Background:
Diabetes is a chronic condition that requires continuous monitoring and management. New technologies, such as **continuous glucose monitors (CGMs)**, offer patients more real-time data about their blood sugar levels. However, real-world data is needed to assess how these technologies perform over time in diverse patient populations, particularly in relation to improving glycemic control and reducing complications.

Application:
An RWE study was launched to assess the real-world impact of CGMs in patients with **Type 2 Diabetes (T2D)** who were not adequately controlled with standard therapies. Data was collected from **EHRs, claims data**, and **patient-reported outcomes** through surveys and wearables tracking daily glucose readings and insulin use.

Findings:
The study demonstrated that the use of CGMs led to significant improvements in **glycemic control** (e.g., reduced HbA1c levels) and a decreased risk of diabetic complications such as retinopathy and nephropathy. Patients using CGMs also reported higher satisfaction with their diabetes management due to the convenience and accuracy of the technology. However, some patients had difficulty adjusting to the device, especially older adults with less experience with digital health tools.

Impact:
The results were used to advocate for the **wider adoption of CGMs** in diabetes management, particularly for patients with **poor glycemic control**. This case highlights how RWE can accelerate the integration of new technologies into routine practice and improve outcomes for patients with chronic diseases like diabetes.

Case Study 10: Rwe In Cancer Treatment Personalization

Background:
Cancer treatment is becoming increasingly personalized, with targeted therapies and immunotherapies being developed based on genetic biomarkers. However, the efficacy of these therapies in the real world, especially across diverse populations, needs to be thoroughly evaluated to ensure that treatment plans align with patients' specific needs.

Application:
A new **targeted cancer therapy** for **non-small cell lung cancer (NSCLC)** was approved based on clinical trials showing efficacy in patients with specific genetic mutations. However, the real-world effectiveness of this therapy, especially in patients with different genetic profiles or comorbid conditions, required further assessment.

RWE was collected through **oncology registries**, **EHRs**, and **genomic data** to evaluate the treatment's effectiveness in the general population. The study focused on outcomes like progression-free survival, overall survival, and quality of life in a cohort of real-world patients with **NSCLC** who received the targeted therapy.

Findings:
The RWE study revealed that the targeted therapy significantly improved survival outcomes for patients with the genetic mutation identified in clinical trials. However, patients with **comorbid conditions** (e.g., cardiovascular disease) had a slightly higher risk of treatment-related complications. Additionally, a subgroup of patients with **minority ethnic backgrounds** showed better-than-expected outcomes, which had not been fully explored in clinical trials.

Impact:
The findings led to further **genomic profiling** being recommended for all patients with NSCLC, even those without a prior diagnosis of the identified genetic mutation. The study also prompted the **refinement of treatment guidelines** to address the needs of patients with comorbid conditions, ensuring that the new therapy was used appropriately in diverse real-world populations.

APPENDICES

Appendix 1: Glossary Of Terms In Real-World Evidence And Data

1. **Real-World Data (RWD)**: Data collected from various sources outside of traditional clinical trials, such as electronic health records (EHRs), insurance claims data, patient registries, and wearable devices, reflecting actual patient experiences.

2. **Real-World Evidence (RWE)**: Evidence derived from the analysis of RWD that is used to support clinical decision-making, regulatory approvals, and healthcare policies.

3. **Propensity Score Matching (PSM)**: A statistical technique used to reduce bias in observational studies by matching patients with similar characteristics (propensity scores) from different treatment groups.

4. **Cohort Study**: An observational study where a group of individuals with common characteristics is followed over time to observe outcomes or compare different treatments.

5. **Case-Control Study**: A study that compares individuals with a specific condition (cases) to those without the condition (controls) to identify factors that may have contributed to the disease.

6. **Cross-Sectional Study**: A study that examines data from a population at a single point in time to evaluate relationships between exposures and outcomes.

7. **Survival Analysis**: A set of statistical methods used to

analyze the time until an event of interest occurs, often used to evaluate treatment effectiveness or mortality rates.

8. **Adaptive Trial**: A clinical trial design that allows for modifications to the trial procedures (e.g., dosing, sample size) based on interim results.

9. **Patient-Reported Outcomes (PROs)**: Health outcomes directly reported by the patient, without interpretation by clinicians or anyone else. These often include symptoms, quality of life, and treatment satisfaction.

10. **Machine Learning (ML)**: A type of artificial intelligence (AI) that involves training algorithms to identify patterns and make predictions based on large datasets, commonly used in RWE to analyze complex data and identify trends.

11. **Data Imputation**: A statistical method for handling missing data by predicting and filling in missing values based on observed data.

12. **Selection Bias**: A type of bias that occurs when the participants selected for a study are not representative of the broader population, which can skew results.

13. **Confounding**: When an external factor influences both the treatment and the outcome, making it difficult to establish a causal relationship.

14. **Health Technology Assessment (HTA)**: The process of evaluating the properties, effects, and impact of healthcare interventions, which can include RWE to inform healthcare policies and reimbursement decisions.

15. **Regulatory Submission**: The formal process through which pharmaceutical companies provide data and evidence to regulatory bodies like the FDA or EMA for the approval of new treatments.

Appendix 2: Recommended Tools And Software For Rwe Research

The following tools and software are commonly used in RWE research to collect, analyze, and visualize data. They can help ensure the quality and integrity of RWD and support the statistical analysis required for RWE studies.

1. **Statistical Software**:
    - **R**: An open-source programming language and software environment used for statistical computing and graphics. It is highly flexible and widely used in RWE research for data analysis, modeling, and visualization.
    - **SAS**: A software suite used for advanced analytics, business intelligence, and data management. SAS is popular for clinical trials and healthcare data analysis.
    - **SPSS**: A software package used for statistical analysis, including descriptive statistics, regression modeling, and data visualization.
    - **Stata**: A software tool for data analysis, particularly in epidemiology and social sciences, widely used for handling large datasets and performing complex statistical analyses.
2. **Data Management Tools**:
    - **RedCap**: A secure, web-based application for building and managing data collection forms. It is commonly used in academic research and clinical settings for collecting patient data.

- **SQL (Structured Query Language)**: A standard programming language for managing and querying relational databases, essential for handling large datasets in RWE research.
- **OpenClinica**: A clinical data management system used for collecting and managing data in clinical trials and other research studies.

3. **Data Cleaning and Transformation**:
    - **Trifacta**: A data wrangling tool designed to clean and transform raw data into a more usable format for analysis. It is especially useful when working with large, complex datasets.
    - **Alteryx**: A data blending and advanced analytics platform that integrates data from multiple sources and prepares it for analysis.

4. **Visualization Tools**:
    - **Tableau**: A powerful tool for creating interactive visualizations and dashboards. It is useful for presenting RWE findings in a clear and engaging manner.
    - **Power BI**: A business analytics tool from Microsoft that enables the creation of visual reports and dashboards. It is commonly used in healthcare settings to analyze and visualize RWD.

5. **Machine Learning and AI Tools**:
    - **TensorFlow**: An open-source framework for building and training machine learning models, often used in RWE for predictive analytics and pattern recognition in large

datasets.

- **Scikit-learn**: A machine learning library in Python that provides simple and efficient tools for data mining and data analysis, including algorithms for classification, regression, and clustering.

Appendix 3: Key Regulatory Guidelines And Frameworks For Rwe

Regulatory agencies play a critical role in the approval and adoption of RWE studies in drug development, healthcare interventions, and policy decisions. The following are key regulatory frameworks and guidelines for RWE research:

1. **U.S. Food and Drug Administration (FDA):**
    - **FDA Framework for Real-World Evidence**: The FDA has outlined a framework for integrating RWE into regulatory decision-making, including its use for post-market surveillance, regulatory approvals, and labeling updates. The FDA's guidance emphasizes the importance of quality RWD sources, robust study designs, and statistical rigor.
    - **21st Century Cures Act**: This legislation encourages the use of RWE in drug development and regulatory processes. It supports the use of RWE for evaluating the safety and effectiveness of medical products, especially in rare diseases and post-marketing surveillance.
2. **European Medicines Agency (EMA):**
    - **EMA's Reflection Paper on Real-World Evidence**: This document provides guidelines for using RWE in regulatory processes, emphasizing its role in the post-market phase, pharmacovigilance, and health technology assessments.
    - **EUnetHTA**: The European Network for Health Technology Assessment supports

the integration of RWE into HTA processes, helping guide reimbursement and healthcare decision-making.

3. **Health Canada**:
    - **Guidance on the Use of Real-World Data and Evidence in Regulatory Decision Making**: This document outlines the framework for using RWE in drug submissions, focusing on data quality, study design, and how RWE can complement traditional clinical trials.

4. **International Society for Pharmacoeconomics and Outcomes Research (ISPOR)**:
    - **Good Research Practices for RWE**: ISPOR has established guidelines for conducting high-quality RWE studies, covering aspects such as study design, data sources, and statistical methodologies.

5. **World Health Organization (WHO)**:
    - **WHO Global Initiative for Evidence-Based Medicine**: WHO encourages the use of RWE to inform healthcare policy, especially in resource-limited settings, and advocates for strengthening national health systems through the use of robust real-world data.

Appendix 4: Further Reading And Resources

For those looking to deepen their knowledge of Real-World Evidence research, the following resources provide in-depth information and insights:

1. **Books**:
    - *Real-World Evidence: The Role of Data and*

Evidence in Healthcare Decision-Making by John P. A. Ioannidis and others.

- *Practical Guide to Conducting Clinical Research* by Leslie T. Vasquez.
- *Observational Studies in Epidemiology: Methods and Applications* by Geoffrey R. Norman.

2. **Journals:**
   - *Journal of Comparative Effectiveness Research*: Focuses on RWE and its applications in evaluating healthcare interventions.
   - *Pharmacoepidemiology and Drug Safety*: Publishes studies on drug safety, effectiveness, and pharmacoepidemiology using RWE.
   - *The Journal of Medical Internet Research (JMIR)*: Covers the intersection of healthcare, technology, and RWE, including the use of mobile health apps and wearables in research.

3. **Online Resources:**
   - **FDA's Real-World Evidence Program**: FDA website
   - **ISPOR Real-World Evidence Resources**: ISPOR website
   - **Health Data Management**: HealthDataManagement.com, a comprehensive resource for news and trends in health data and RWE.

4. **Workshops and Webinars:**
   - **ISPOR Conferences**: ISPOR hosts regular workshops and conferences focusing on RWE and health economics.

- **FDA and EMA Webinars**: Both the FDA and EMA offer webinars on the latest RWE guidance and regulations.

ABOUT THE AUTHOR

Dr Essam Abdelhakim

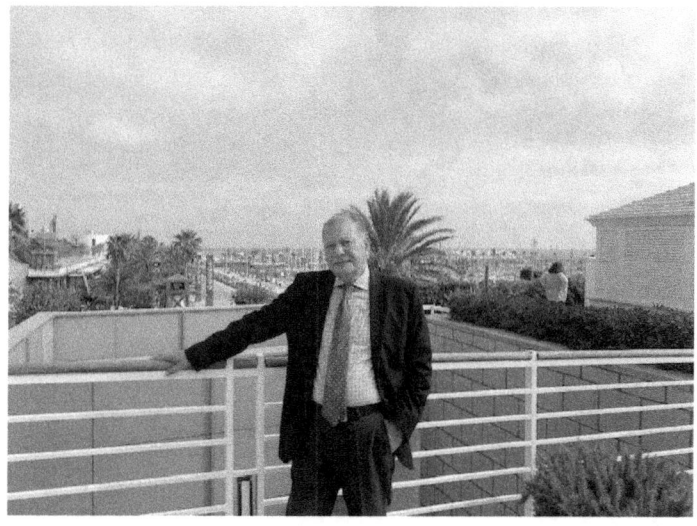

Senior Investigator and Expert in Clinical Research